For Mom,
who gave me her
love of fitness.

STOVER

STOVER By Kat

The Winner Is...   Kathy B

Purrsnikitty   By Kathy Bro

just sniffing around   By Kathy Bro

the **Inside** Story   By Kathy

My Bent Tree   by Kathy Broc

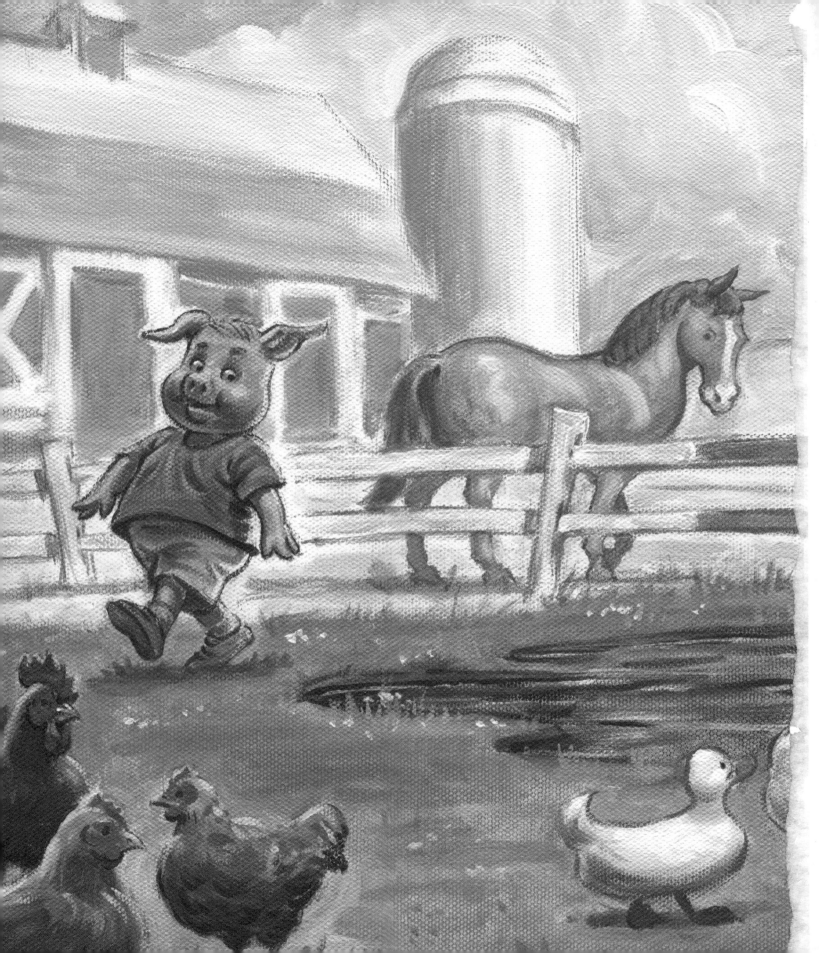

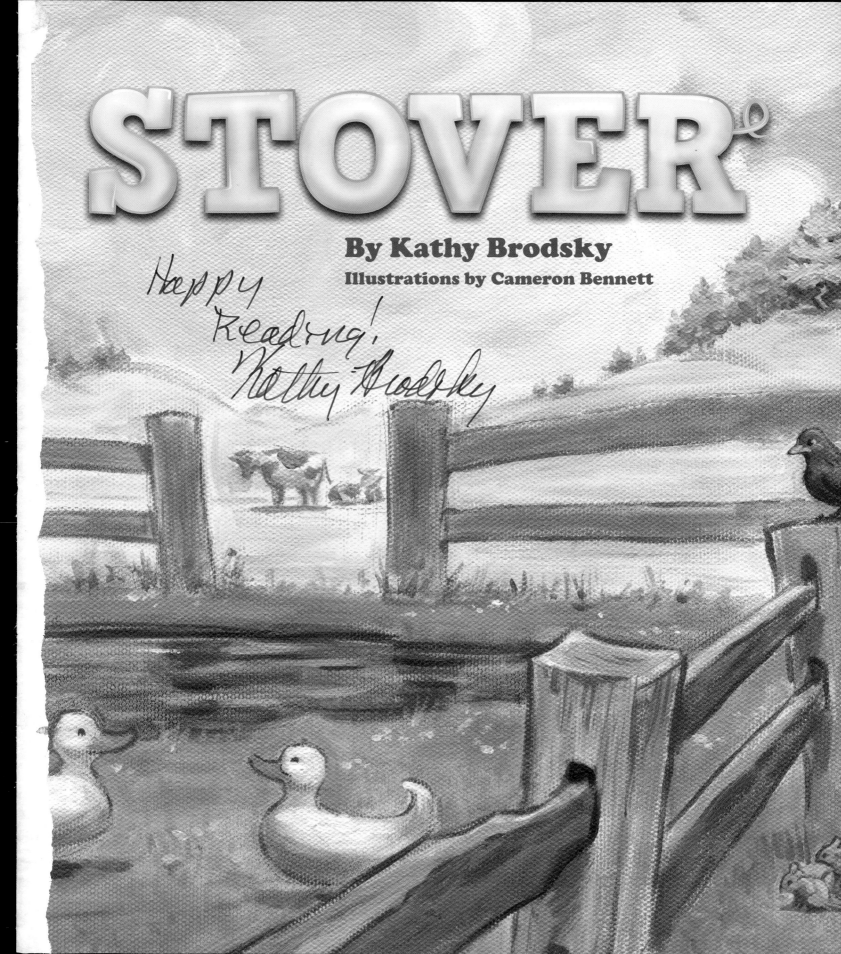

STOVER

By Kathy Brodsky

Illustrations by Cameron Bennett

Happy
Reading!
Kathy Brodsky

My name is Stover.
I'm a neat pig.

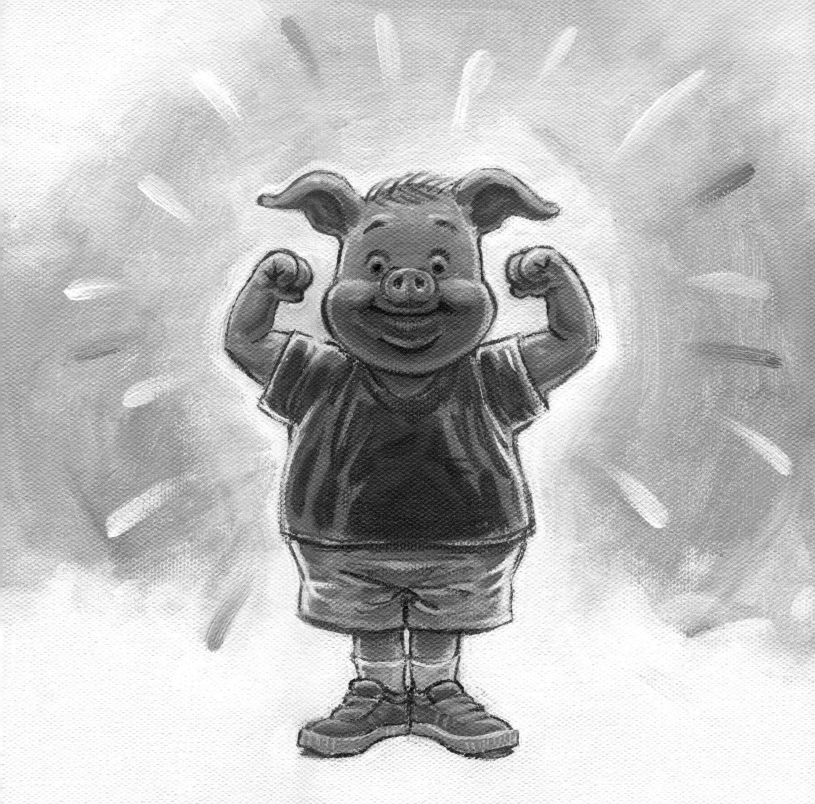

I keep myself healthy
in small ways and big!

I often go stomping
in piles of wet mud.

I **slosh** and then spin—
quickly drop with a thud.

**Once I am finished
I roll around more—**

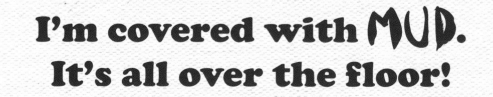

**I'm covered with MUD.
It's all over the floor!**

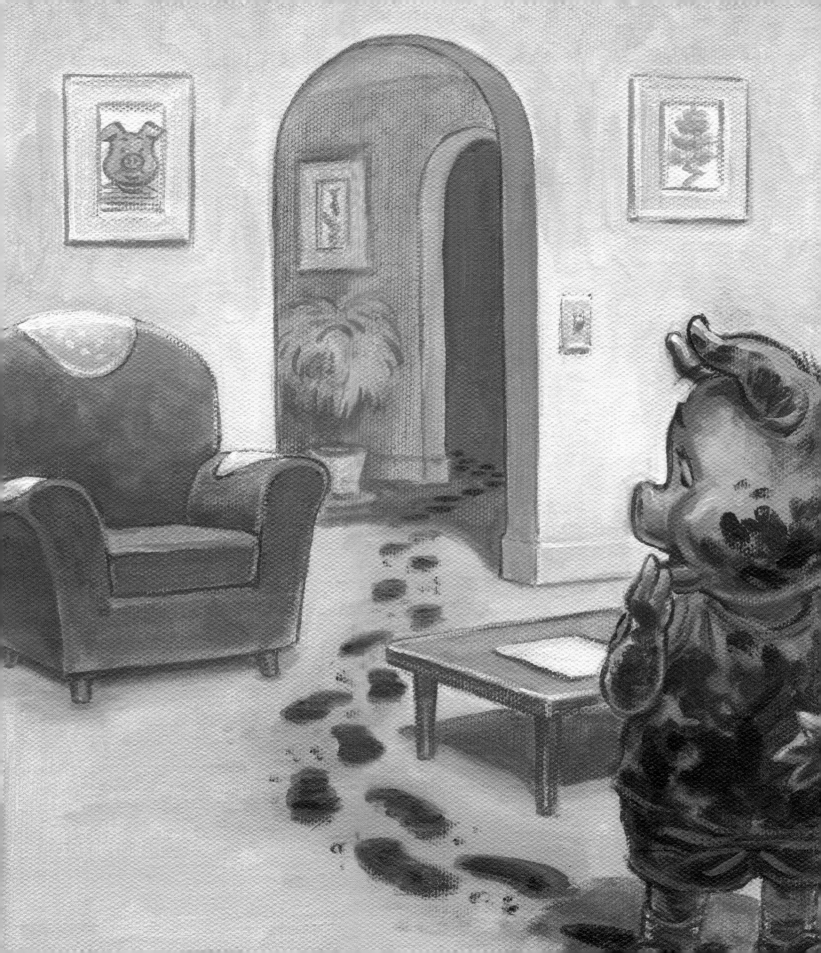

Then I get cleaned up,
I shower and run.
I can't wait to get to
the gym and have fun!

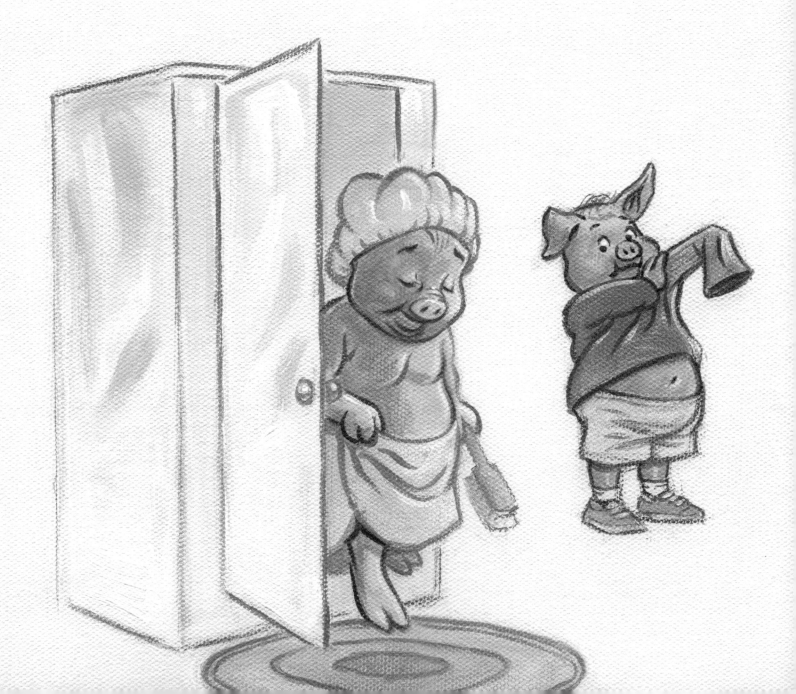

But...

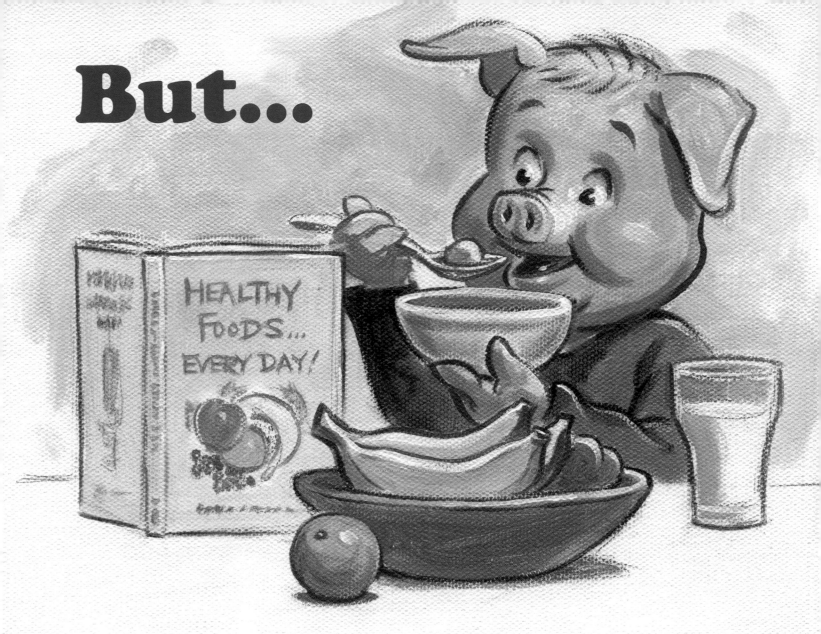

First I eat breakfast—
my oatmeal and fruit
with milk and my fruit juice—
it helps me re-boot!

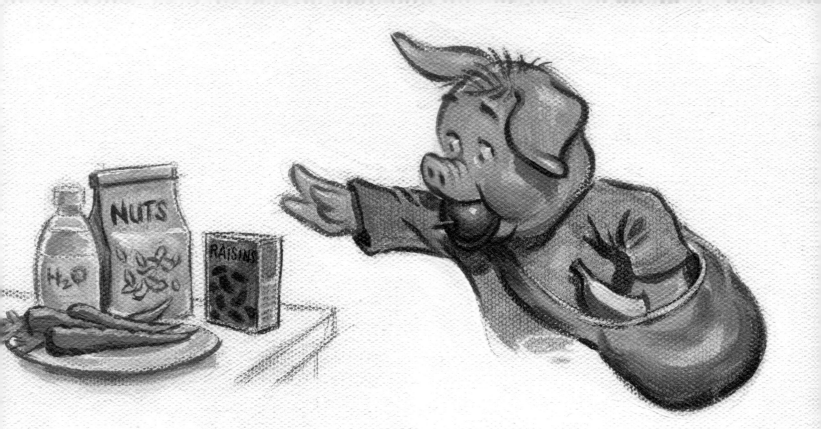

**On my way out the door
I grab some good snacks.**

When I get to the gym
they say, "Hi, glad you're back!"

I use the stair climber,
and drink from a cup.

While watching TV
I climb up and up!

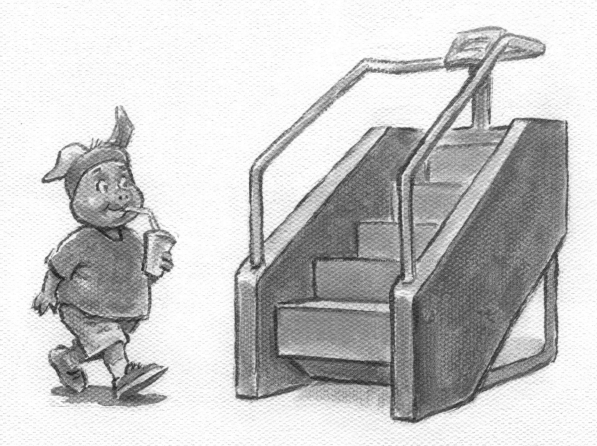

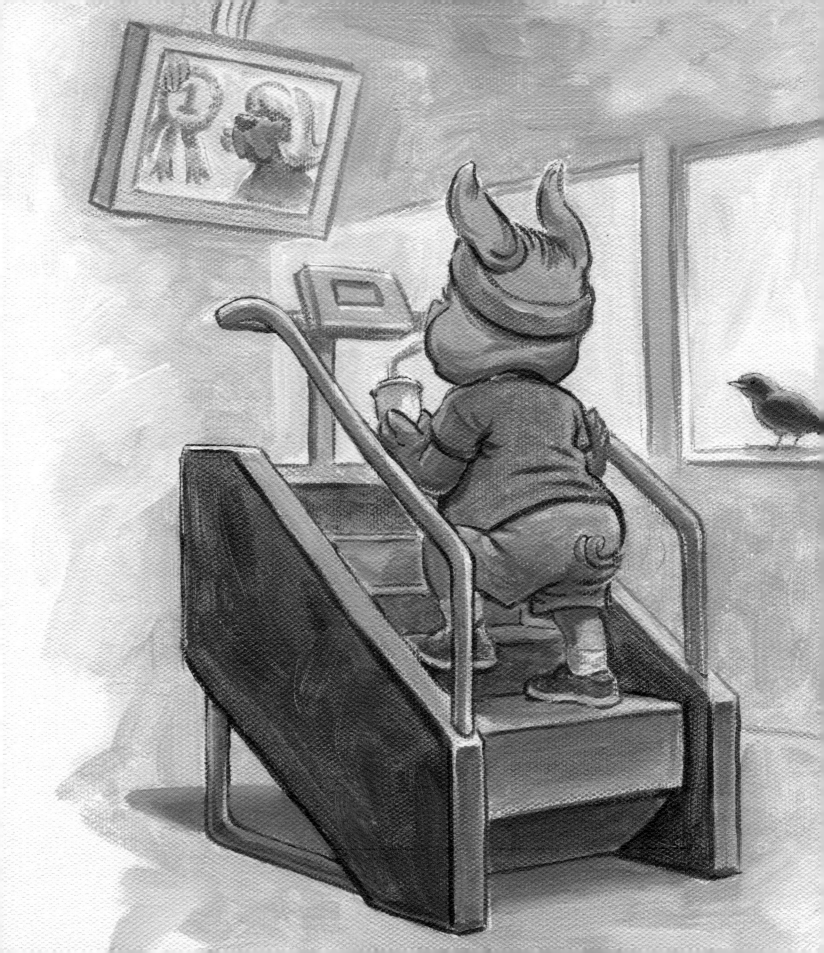

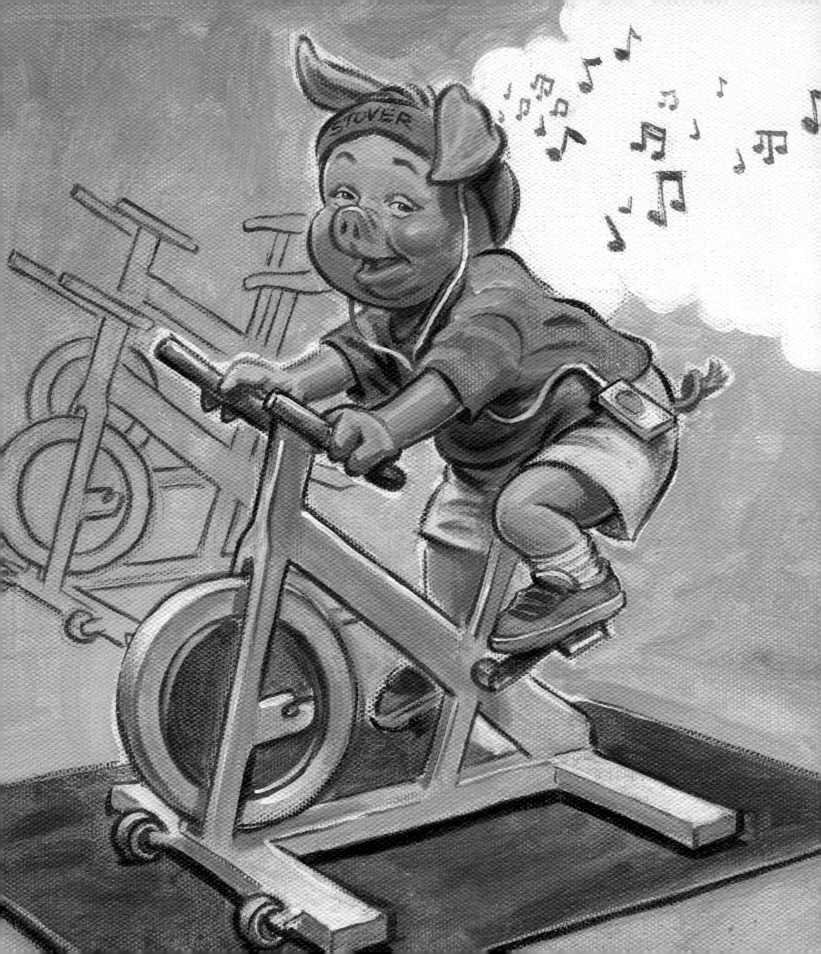

I love to go spinning—
my legs pump quite *FAST*.

I listen to music—
some new hits, some past.

I have a great trainer—
his name is Steve.

He gives me new workouts—
has lots up his sleeve.

I also do yoga—
my body bends well.

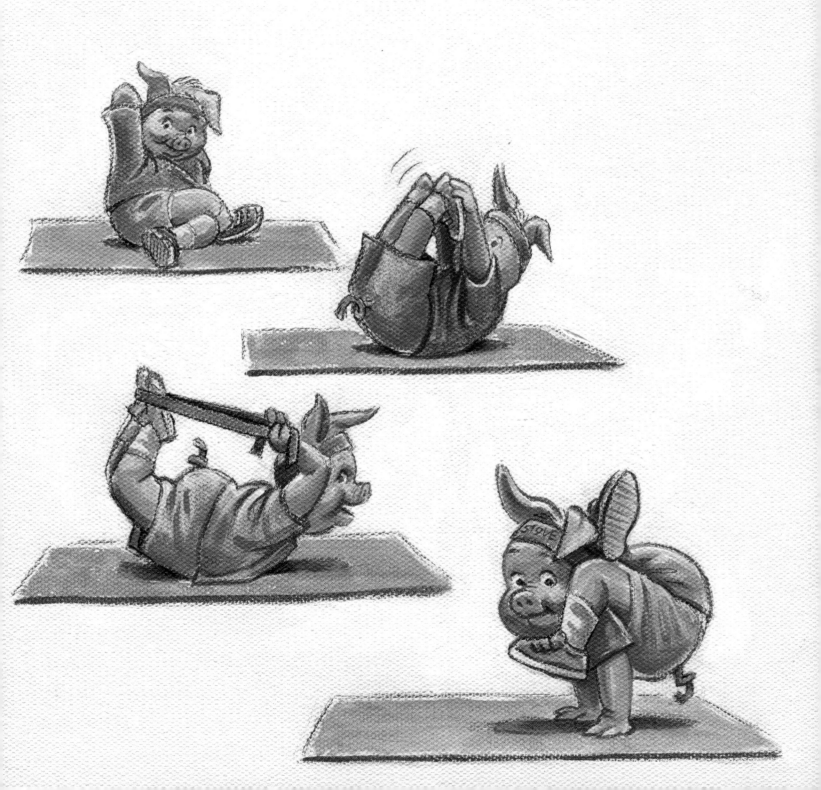

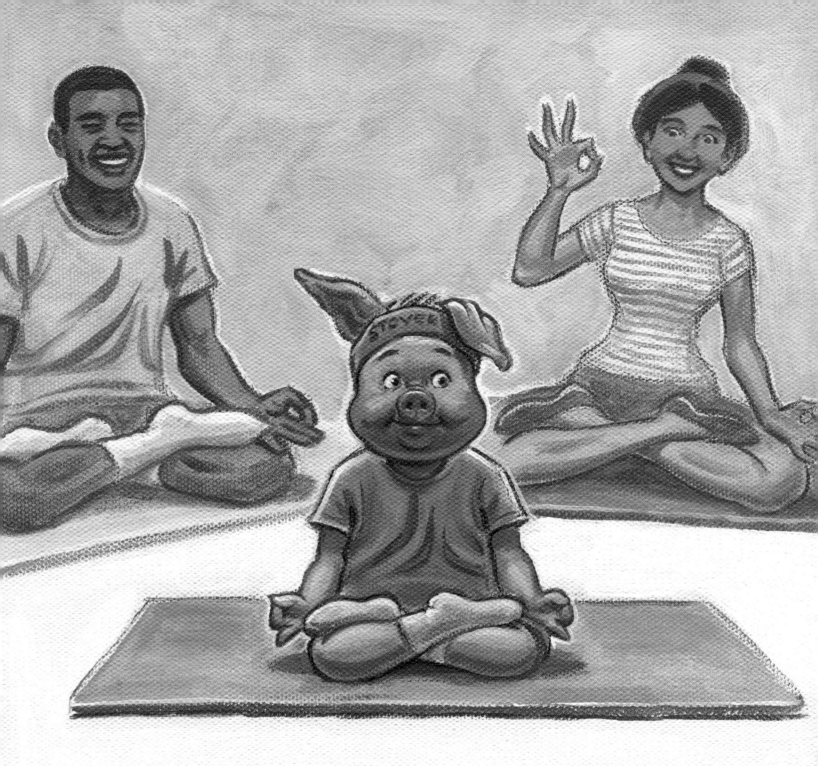

I hold all my poses.
The class thinks I'm swell!

I walk on the treadmill
and talk quite a bit.

My neighbors are friendly.
I'm such a BIG hit!

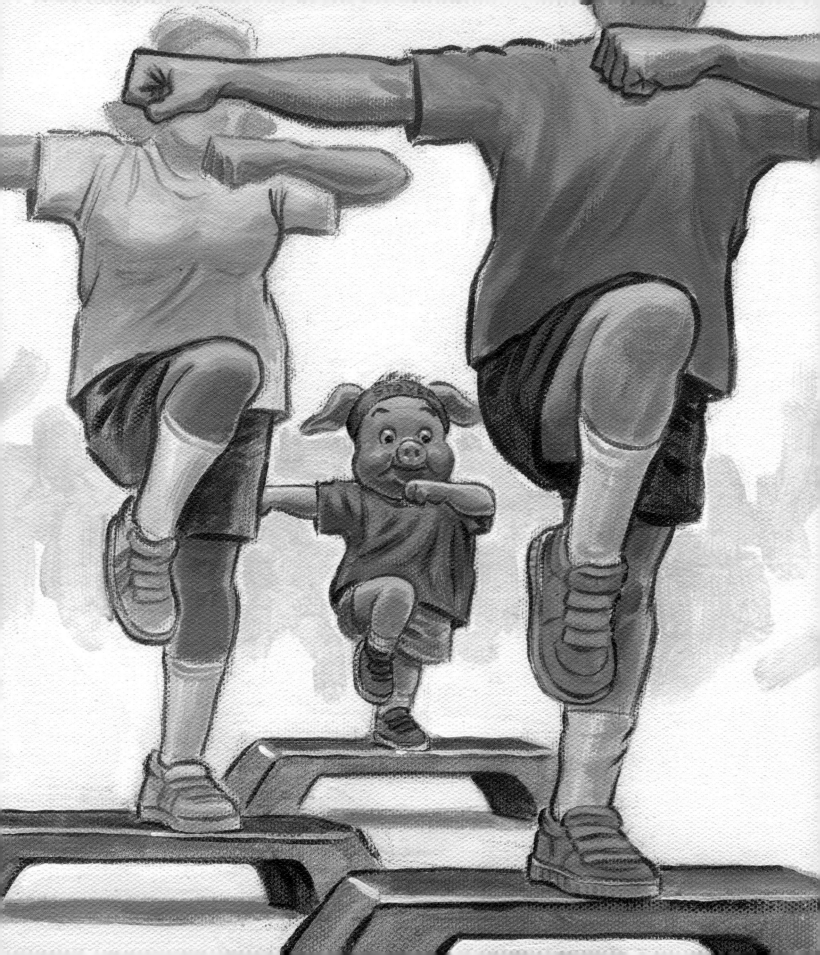

Aerobics is peppy.
It makes me sweat tons.

Sometimes I do step class
which firms up my buns.

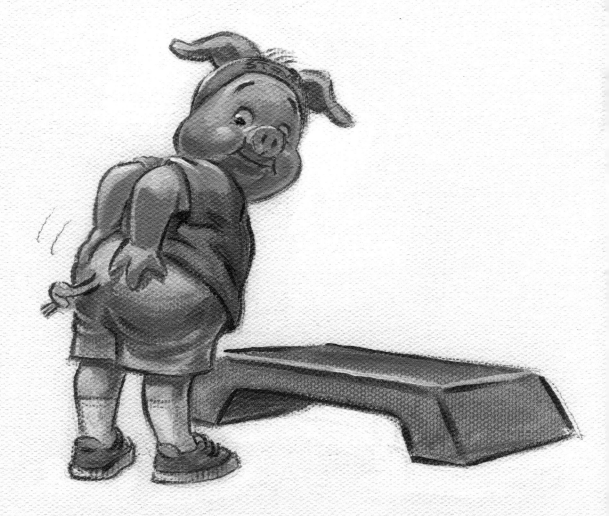

I go to the back room
to **stretch**. It's the best.

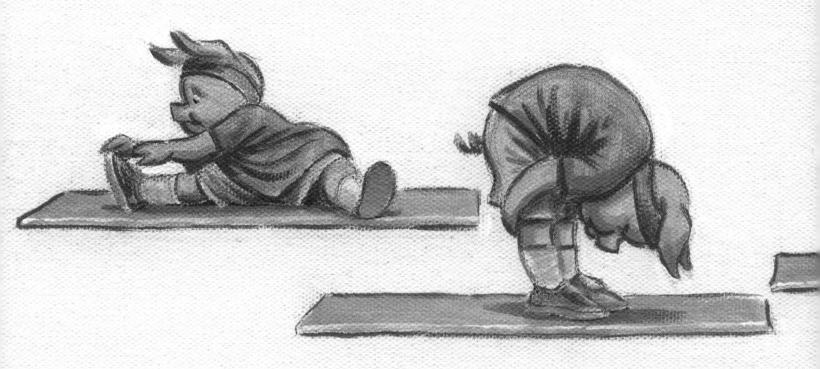

I grab a new mat—
twist, turn—time to rest.

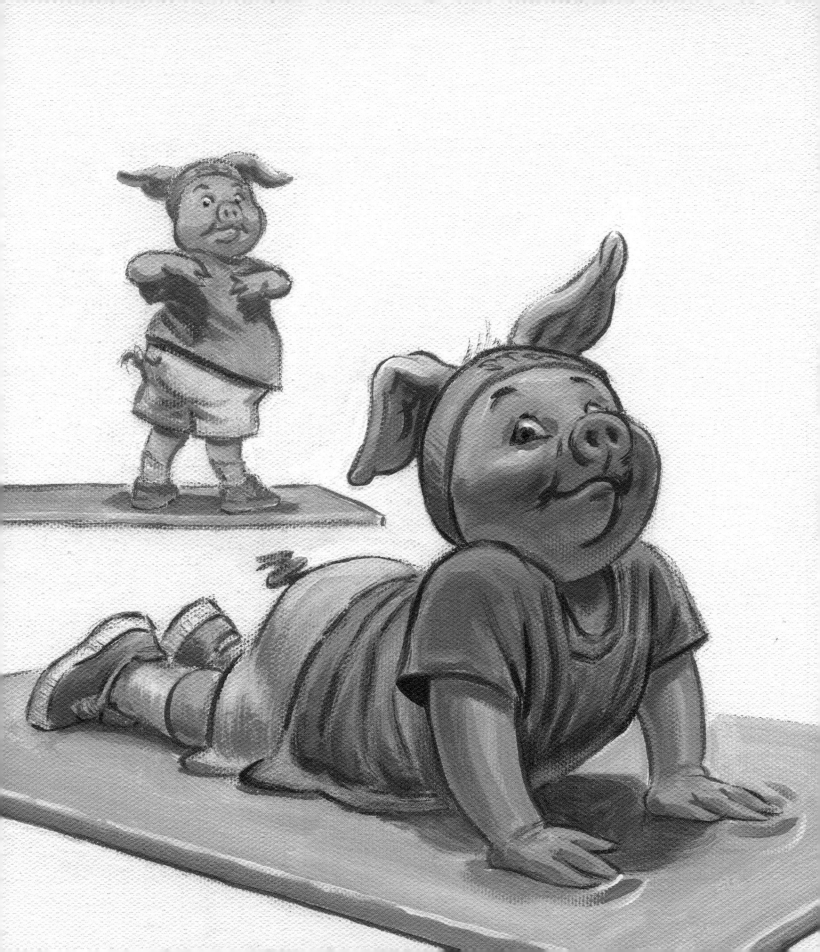

It's fun to swim fast
with goggles and cap.

The swim team has noticed.
They want me for laps!

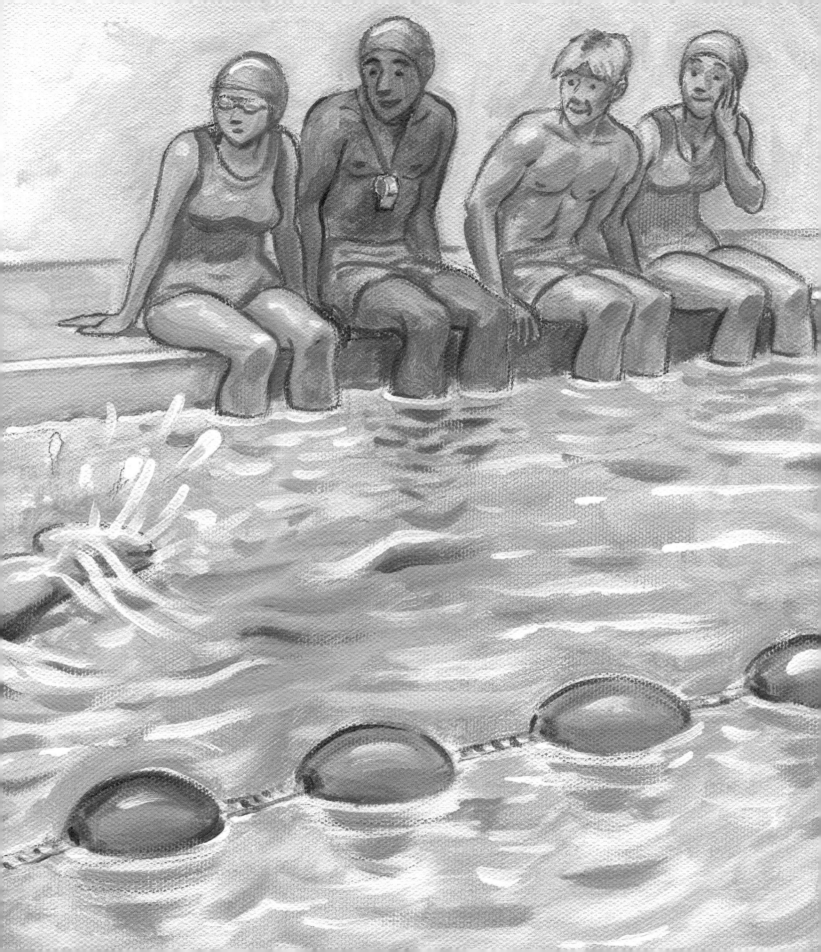

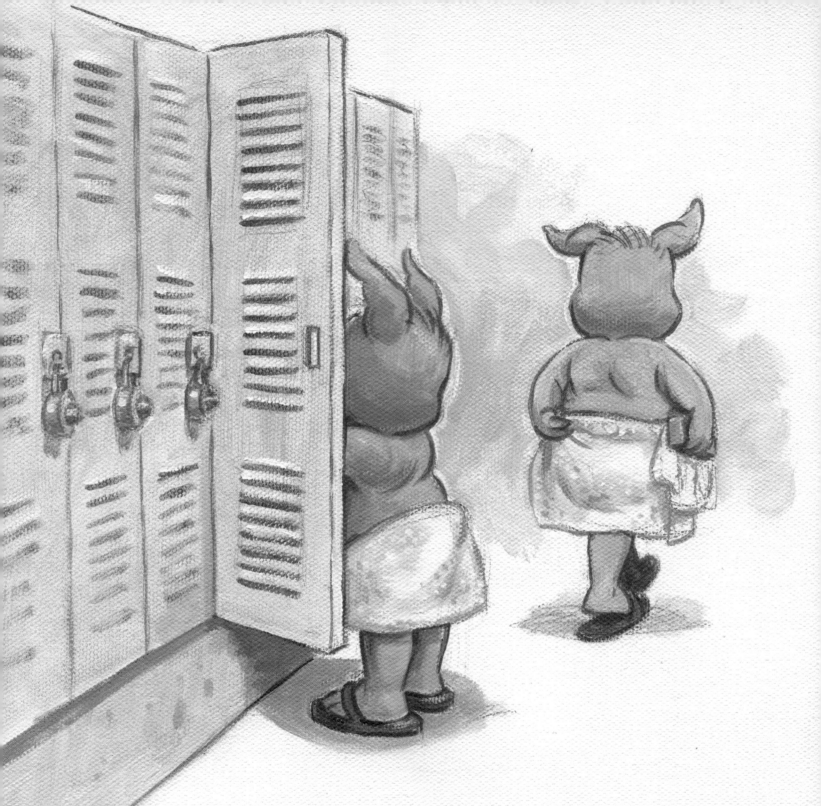

**I'm off to the lockers—
I'm finished with play.**

I shower, change quickly— energized for the day.

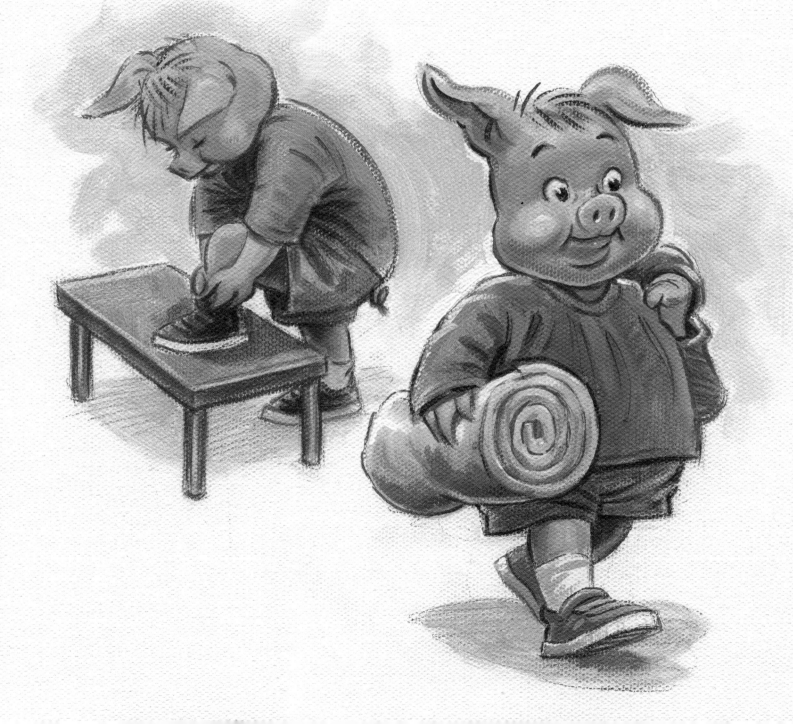

I look in the mirror.
Hooray! I pinch less.

I feel so terrific.
I'm such a success!

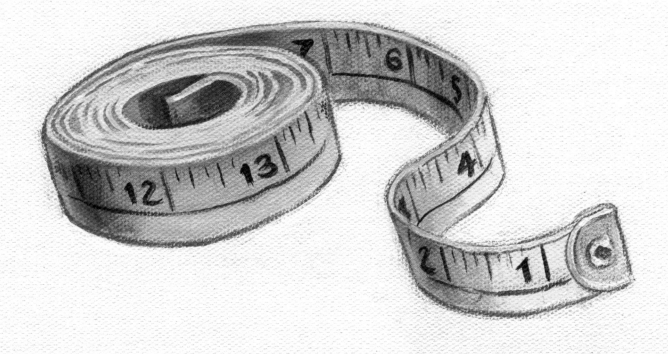

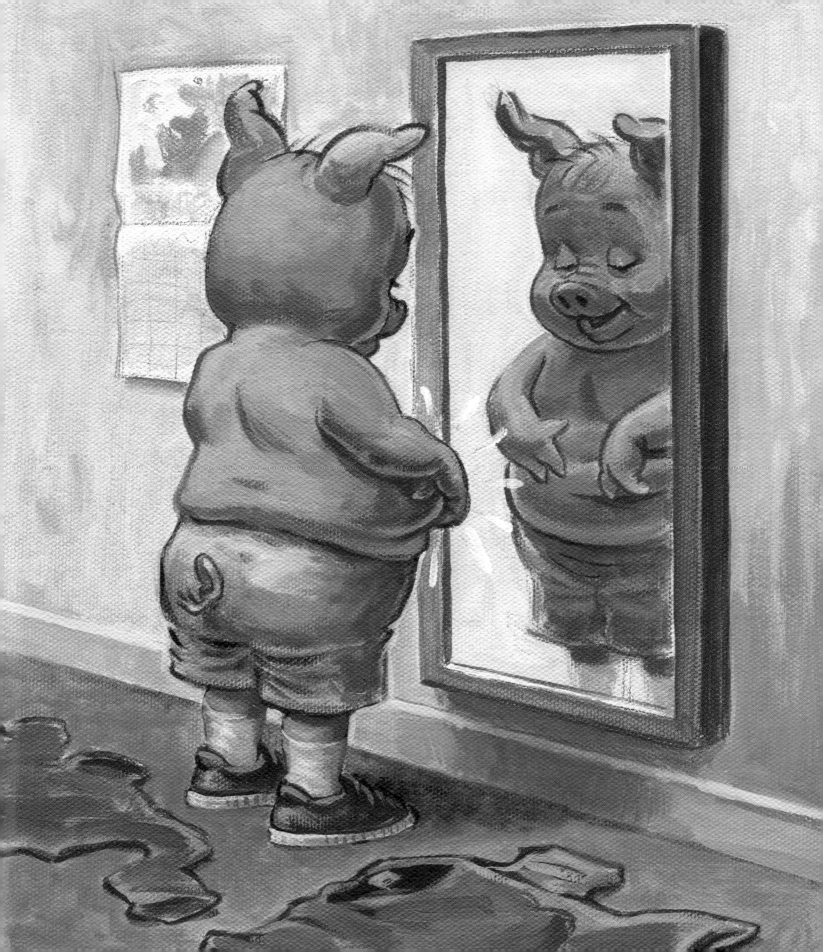

Find *your* way to fitness.
The gym is *my* game!

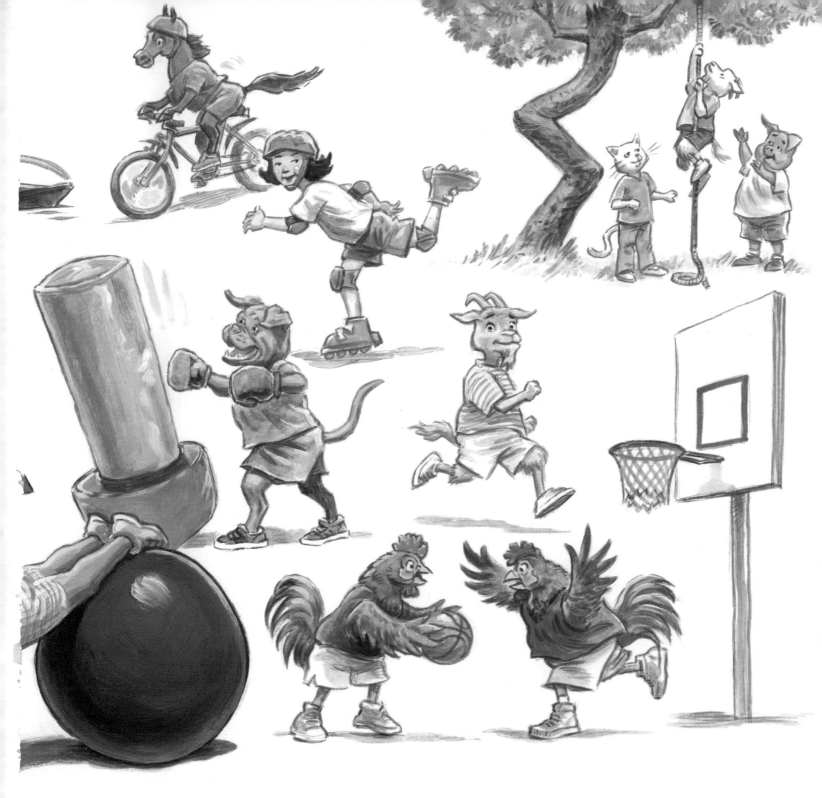

**I love being healthy.
Get fit!! Do the same!!**

FITNESS

- [ ] **1** **What is "good health?"**

- [ ] **2** How can you tell if you're healthy?

- [ ] **3** **How can you tell if you're a good size and weight for a healthy person your age?**
  If you aren't—what can you do about it?

- [ ] **4** In a 24 hour day, how much time do you spend sitting?
  What are you doing when you're sitting?

- [ ] **5** **How many times a week do you have gym class?**
  What types of activities do you do?

- [ ] **6** If your school doesn't have a gym program, why don't they?
  What can you do to get one?

- [ ] **7** **What do you do for exercise or sports when you're not in school?**

- [ ] **8** What kind of fun games or exercises can you make up to "move your body?"

- [ ] **9** **Do your family members exercise?**
  What do they do to stay fit?

FOOD

- [ ] **1** Why is it necessary to eat?

- [ ] **2** What are healthy foods and why are they important?
  What kind of healthy foods do you eat?

- [ ] **3** Why is some food called "junk" food?
  What would happen to your body if you ate only "junk" food?

- [ ] **4** What are the different food groups of The Food Guide Pyramid?
  Give examples of foods found in each.

- [ ] **5** Name the six basic nutrients found in food.
  What does each one do to keep your body healthy?

- [ ] **6** Look at a food label. What kind of information does it give you?

- [ ] **7** What fun, healthy snacks and recipes can you make?

FUNTIVITY!

Write a sentence, story or play, make up a poem, or sing a song about being fit and eating in a healthy way!

Stover is a pig, not a proverbial "fat pig," but a pig who knows how to stay fit and eat healthy foods. After his brief appearance in my book **The Winner Is...** some friends suggested that I write a book about him. After all, pigs are considered among the brightest of farm animals.

Though **Stover** is only a pig, he is bright enough to know how important it is to eat healthy foods—but not too much—and to exercise regularly.

He's plump, but he's fit!

Exercise and good nutrition are keys to being healthy.

Kathy Brodsky

Kathy Brodsky

Thanks SO Much!

Stover is one of the most fit, adorable little pigs you've ever met! Many wonderful people helped bring him to life—especially: Cameron, Julia, Mary, Louise, Kim and Aaron at wedü, Greg, Jeff, Bedford Writers' Group, Marilyn, Steve, Kathy, and the students at Green Acres School.

Publisher's Cataloging-in-Publication
(Provided by Quality Books, Inc.)

Brodsky, Kathy.
    Stover / by Kathy Brodsky ; illustrations by Cameron Bennett.
    p. cm.
    SUMMARY: In this rhyming story, Stover, a pig, eats healthy foods and goes to the gym to stay fit.
    ISBN-13: 978-0-9828529-1-0
    ISBN-10: 0-9828529-1-6

    1. Swine--Juvenile fiction. 2. Nutrition--Juvenile fiction. 3. Physical fitness--Juvenile fiction.
[1. Pigs--Fiction. 2. Nutrition--Fiction. 3. Physical fitness--Fiction. 4. Health--Fiction. 5. Stories in rhyme.]   I. Bennett, Cameron (Cameron D.), ill.
II. Title.

PZ8.3.B782Sto 2011   [E]
            QBI11-600039

Published by Helpingwords
Stover © 2011
Printed in the U.S.A
Printed on recycled paper

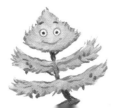

Kathy Brodsky
www.kathybrodsky.com
Manchester, NH 03104
ISBN-13: 978-0-9828529-1-0

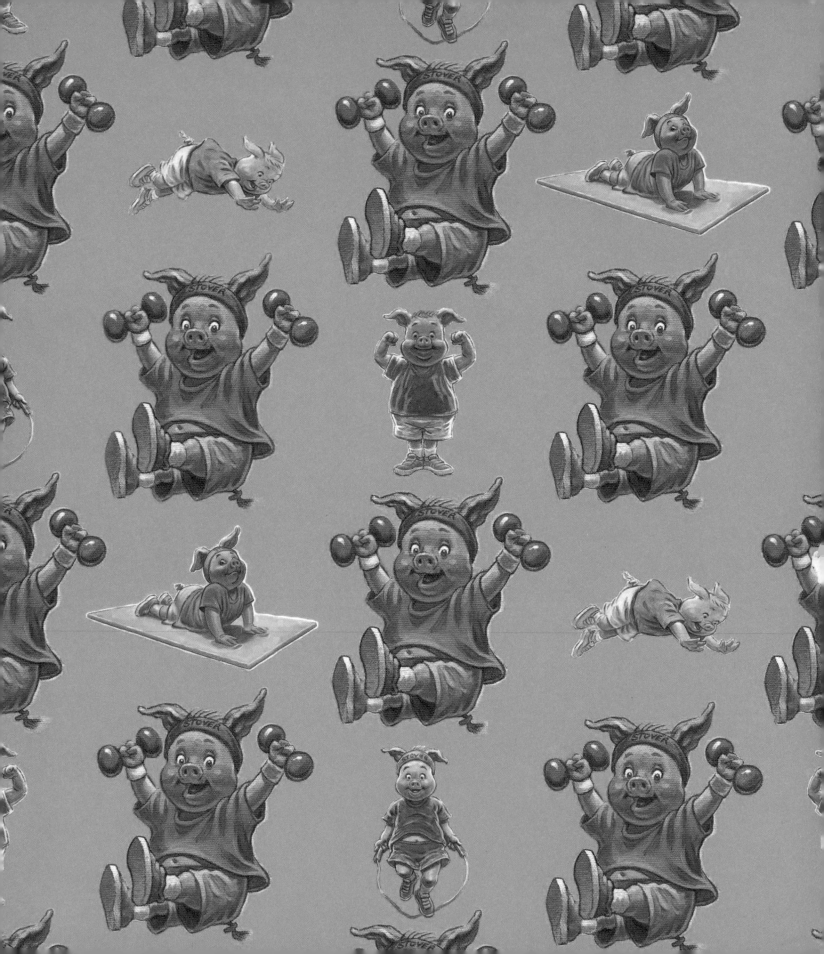